SPECIAL CASES

JONATHAN HULL

Magic Daisy Publishing

First published 2022 by Magic Daisy Publishing

www.magicdaisypublishing.co.uk

Copyright © Magic Daisy Publishing 2022
Text copyright © Jonathan Hull 2022

ISBN 979-8-8136-4132-9

Printed and bound by Amazon

SPECIAL CASES

Content warning: This book contains disturbing and upsetting material, including physical and sexual violence, major trauma, death and suicide. It is intended for adult readers only.

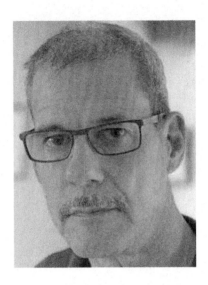

Jonathan was educated at Uppingham School and Birmingham University Medical School, graduating in 1983. He joined the Army and served for 19 years, with postings to Germany and the USA, and operational tours in Northern Ireland, Iraq, Bosnia, Congo and Kosovo. He was parachute trained and provided surgical support for UK Special Forces.

After leaving the Army he was a Consultant Orthopaedic Surgeon at Frimley Park NHS Foundation Trust from 1999-2020, specialising in all aspects of hip and knee surgery as well as trauma management.

Jonathan is married and has four grown-up children and two grandchildren. He has now retired from NHS practice and lives in Norfolk where, as it happens, he grew up. He shoots regularly at Bisley and has represented Hampshire, England and Great Britain.

Foreword

The words 'thank you' just don't seem to cut it, but I will never stop thanking Jonathan Hull, thanking him for saving my life. The odds were most definitely stacked against me (300:1 according to Michael Buerk on the subsequent BBC 999 episode), and he never gave up. Had he not been the consultant on-call on that fateful day in 1998, I believe the outcome would have been very different.

When I returned to Frimley Park Hospital for rehabilitation on the military ward - an offer that was kindly extended during my transfer to Roehampton Burns Unit whilst still in a very critical condition - I said to Jonathan, or Colonel Hull, as I addressed him back then:

'I bet you never actually thought I'd be back here!'.

I will never forget his response:

'I knew from the minute we tried to cut off your clothes in the resus room, that you would survive. On the battlefield when soldiers fight not to have their fatigues cut off, it's always a sure sign that they will pull through'.

Yes, I had that fighting spirit, but I would not be here without such a skilled military consultant.

I am so grateful that we have managed to stay in touch after all these years, and so very honoured to write this foreword. Most people would have watched box sets and gorged on chocolate after having their hip replaced, but not Jonathan, he writes a book!

Louise McOvens
January 2022

CONTENTS

Preface

This book is a collection of short stories. Normally you might expect short stories to be fictional, but these are all totally true and each relates to a particular case that I have been involved with.

Every doctor will have cases that they remember as being either funny, sad, poignant or just plain weird. I don't expect mine are especially different or unique, but to me they are special.

I have tried to relate them with some humour, some humility and always with respect. These tales are about real people and their troubles that I had the privilege to become entangled with and sometimes to help during my military career and in the years that followed.

My friend and orthopaedic colleague, Hugh Chissell, has also kindly donated a memorable tale (Frank) to include in this collection.

Where possible I have obtained permission from the patients I have included. When that has not been possible, I have changed names to protect their privacy.

Louise and the fence

The case I am about to relate is the most dramatic and unforgettable of my whole career. It tells the story from Day 1 in 1998 right up until the present day, as luck would have it.

Louise was 18 years old in 1998, and like many teenagers she had a busy social life. And a car. So, not surprisingly, her car-less friends would sometimes lean on her to take them places. It was no bother because she loved her little car and loved driving, and if she had to be the one who didn't drink, that was no problem. Louise was happy to be a 'nominated driver' for her mates. Right up until that fateful day in January 1998.

They had all been dancing somewhere in South London. Afterwards Louise and her friends had tried sleeping in a friend's flat but they only had coats to lie on and in the end they decided to go home. Louise was stone-cold sober but was maybe a little tired. No matter, she was 18 and full of life so driving after being up most of the night, especially the short hop back to Farnham, wouldn't be a problem for her. Two cups of coffee and she was good to go!

So there they were, Louise and her two mates, trundling along the M3 in the early morning sunshine. There was music on the radio, but one of the guys wanted it turned down a bit as it was keeping him awake. Louise was driving carefully, not going fast – well, to be honest, her precious little car wasn't able to speed much with three on board – and inside it was nice and warm and quiet. Not much traffic on a Saturday morning and a clear road. Oh dear.

The next thing Louise remembers is crashing down the slight embankment beside the motorway, and seeing a wooden fence in her way. The car smashed through the fence and came to a juddering halt up against a tree. For a moment it was all quiet apart from the hiss of steam coming from the bonnet and the birds squawking in anger at being disturbed. There was motorway noise in the background but it was just a hum really.

Then everyone was shouting and screaming all at once. The boys managed to scramble out of the passenger door, helped by a passing lorry driver, Jim Hodder, and Bob Waite, a taxi driver, who had straightaway stopped to help. What a mess! 'Come on Louise, get out!' they screamed, 'it might blow up!' The driver's door was jammed and Bob had to smash the window to reach in and turn off the ignition, cutting his hand in the process.

As her friends looked on in horror, Louise began to smell burning. There was smoke now coming from under the bonnet and into the wheel wells. Then flames began to flicker and, after a moment, she realised in horror that her jeans were on fire. Stuck in her seat, she was terrified she was going to burn to death.

Louise knew she needed to get out and she really wanted to, but try as she might, she just couldn't seem to move. She seemed to be trapped in her seat for some reason and although she was pushing with her legs, her bottom just wouldn't shift.

It turned out that a long piece of 4x2 inch wooden panel from the fence had gone in through the front wheel arch when the car crashed through, somehow passing through the seat and then into the back of her thigh, very close to her hip. It went on through her pelvis and lower abdomen and finally exited her lower back, wedging itself into the driver's seat behind her. It was one of those freak occurrences that could never be repeated. It was clear there was no possibility of pulling the post out, and doing so would have killed her anyway.

'Water!, we need water!' someone shouted. But there was none. Jim realised that there were wet leaves everywhere left over after the Autumn fall and he and Bob, who was a former fireman, quickly scooped some up and pushed them through the driver's window onto Louise's legs and feet. More leaves followed and they started to smother the flames. Very probably this one desperate act is what really saved her life. *(Both Jim and Bob needed treatment for smoke inhalation and burns to their hands.)*

It all got a little confusing after that. A fire engine arrived and a passing emergency doctor (Paul Rees), and paramedics. The fire was put out and Louise was given IV fluids and oxygen. Louise remembers asking them not to damage her little car but the only way to get her out was to dismantle the car around her.

Very carefully, the firemen took off the roof and sides of the car using power-saws and other enormous tools with great delicacy, ensuring that there was no further injury to Louise's legs and trunk. At last, the post was cut, both under her leg and behind her back, so that she could be lifted out onto a stretcher. Incredibly there wasn't much bleeding - on the outside at least; Louise remained fully conscious throughout the whole terrifying ordeal, and can remember feeling the vibrations from the saw as it cut through the post. Then it was into an ambulance and 'blues and twos' to the nearest hospital....

...which is where I joined the story.

In early 1998 I had only been a consultant for about a year. I had had plenty of trauma experience during my training, including a year in a US trauma hospital, so was reasonably competent. That particular Saturday morning I was on the golf course as the hospital was quiet and the Specialist Registrar, Anthony, was extremely senior and was himself waiting for an imminent consultant appointment.

He called me on my mobile. 'You have GOT to come and see what has just arrived in A&E' he said, slightly breathlessly. 'What, like now?' I queried, as I still had three holes to go.

'Can't you cope?' I asked, in that way which really means 'I am far too senior now to go anywhere in a hurry'. But he did mean it, and I duly went in a hurry, as requested.

Imagine the scene. Packed resus room, bodies everywhere (medics not patients). At the centre of which lies a young female on her side on a trolley, looking rather singed around the edges, soaking wet, and with a bloody great piece of wood sticking up in the air from the back of her right leg.

Stay calm, I said to myself. Just another trauma case. They all do well, etc. Start with the basics - airway: clear, she's talking. Bleeding: not so much. Circulation: hmm, maybe not so good, and not likely to get any better when you take that big twig out is it?

Right, make a plan. We need a general surgeon to deal with the intra-abdominal damage. As luck would have it the general surgical consultant was at the opposite end of his career and was due to retire within weeks. He and I had a chat and he deferred to my recent trauma and military experience, suggesting he might 'take a quick look' in theatre and then let me get on with extracting the fence post. Being military, I counter-suggested that his 'quick look' should be a full laparotomy to secure the main vessels, check for internal organ damage and only after that would anybody be pulling the foreign body out. There was slight tension at this point, young buck v senior surgeon, but he got the message well enough.

I won't go into all the gory details but suffice it to say, Operation Fence Post Removal took a good six hours. There inevitably was intra-abdominal damage and Louise would go on to need a colostomy for a year afterwards. There was total severance of her right sciatic nerve and this would ultimately need reconstruction by Professor Rolfe Birch at the Royal National Orthopaedic Hospital, Stanmore *(Louise was only the 3rd patient worldwide to have this done)*. There were terrible circumferential burns around both legs and she underwent multiple skin grafts at Queen Mary's, Roehampton in the year that followed.

But what *really* vexed us on the day, was the 6 inch nail that appeared from the x-ray to be stuck in the fence post, somewhere deep inside her pelvis. There was no way we could knock the post out with that in there as it would have caused unimaginable damage on the way. What to do? Nothing in the textbooks on that one and nothing in my experience bank to refer to. All I could think of was to try and get around the post, up into the pelvis through the leg wound, and bend the nail. Which is exactly what we did, although where the strength to bend a 6 inch nail came from I have no idea. With one of us banging from behind with a hammer, and one of us trying to protect the soft tissues from below, Anthony and I slowly managed to push/pull that oversized splinter out of our patient. Fortunately there was no blood vessel damage inside, and once we had picked all the bits of wood, leaves and other rubbish out, we were able to pack the wounds, fore and aft, dress the burns and get the

'Hell out of Dodge' (as we used to say in Baltimore after a long case).

Job done. For now at least. Or so I thought. I wandered onto ITU an hour or so later to see how Louise was doing. It was late in the evening and I hadn't had the energy to change out of my scrubs by then. 'Please could I speak to her parents?' I was asked, 'they are in the relatives room.' Of course. Parents? The *whole extended family* was packed in there by then, maybe 15 or 20 anxious faces looked up at me when I went in, still a bit dazed. It turned out Louise was the baby of a lovely big family from Crondall, and, as it happened, they were all free to visit that evening. The resultant cross-examination I underwent for the next 30 minutes was probably more stressful than the operation had been. It was certainly harder than any professional viva I had gone through in my training.

These lovely people, who clearly adored Louise, needed to hear that she was going to be OK, and by that I mean back to full working order within a very short time. Having to explain what the injuries were, how badly she had been burned, how precarious the next few days and weeks would be, was very difficult and stressful. For me.

One can only imagine how hard it must have been for them to hear. I knew I had to give them hope but not pretend things would ever be the same again. These were still very much life-threatening injuries and there was no certainty she would survive at this point. If she did, then she was going to be challenged with significant disabilities and might not remain fully intact, as her legs were really badly injured.

Of course, I didn't know then what I do now.

Louise doesn't do 'failure' or 'giving up' or 'I can't'. If she had died on the table in theatre I am quite sure she would have self-willed herself back to life again. She is quite the most remarkable individual I have ever had the privilege to help.

Suffice it to say, she went on to make the most complete recovery one could ever have imagined. She overcame it all and she and her husband set up a kite-surfing school in Cornwall. Even when 23 years later her right foot had to be amputated due to chronic compartment syndrome which had been masked by the original burns, she put on her bouncy prosthesis and you guessed it, got back in the sea again!

We have stayed in touch throughout and I have recently had the pleasure to help sort out her Mum's dodgy knee and hip joints, operations that are significantly less stressful than taking a fence post out of a pelvis.

Louise looked a little surprised when I told her recently that she had been the defining case of my career.

But it's true.

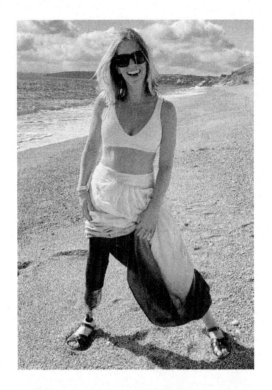

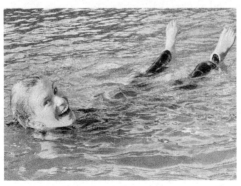

Louise back in action in 2021

Now how did that get in there?

In 1990, I found myself working in Belize, Central America. I was in the Army then and Belize was considered a prime posting for junior surgeons. It may not have been quite so ideal for the soldiers and their families to have a relatively inexperienced surgeon in post, but hey, 'You're in the Army now' and in extremis, there was always a Lear jet to Miami.

Belize was a fascinating country with a population of around 400,000. Situated on the Caribbean coast, between Mexico and Guatemala, I would call it 'Third World (light)' really with a mix of quite sophisticated residential areas in Belize City contrasting with mud-huts in the rural jungle villages. The Mayan Indian population in the South were in contrast to a large Mennonite community in the North, both of which had very little or no medical facilities. On the coast there were tourist resorts catering for diving and other watersports and these were busy during the dry periods. One in particular, Journey's End, was a regular weekend getaway for the RAF contingent in Belize and if you were very good, they would sometimes take you with them in their nice helicopter.

I wanted to explore the country as much as possible during my three months posting and one of the best ways was to take my team to various hospitals and clinics around the country and offer up our services. We travelled either by Land Rover, or helicopter when we could get one, both north and south, finding a warm welcome wherever we turned up.

The Amish were a gentle and gracious people who appreciated our visits and we did what we could using field surgical equipment to perform simple ops such as vasectomies, hernias and even one gall-bladder removal. Mennonites originated in Germany and are very religious and practise extreme pacifism. They travelled across the world, first to North America and then migrated south, often being subjected to violence and intimidation to which they cannot respond due to their beliefs. As a result, they are easy targets for robbery, and worse, and it is very hard to appreciate why they feel they cannot fight back.

The Mayans were delightful colourful people as well, and they insisted on feeding us in return for what little medical help we were providing. This proved very entertaining at times and particularly so watching my team, squatting on the floor of a mud hut doing their best to eat a chicken that 30 minutes earlier had been running around under their feet!

There was an established and regular visit to Belmopan which was a medium sized town/city in the centre of the country, with its own hospital. It wasn't exactly like a NHS hospital but it did have an operating theatre, albeit with a large hole in the wall out to the street. It was safe to do minor ops in there, using both local and general anaesthesia.

I was just finishing up a morning operating list when they asked me if I would see one extra patient who was in trouble in the small A&E department. 'Sure,' I said, 'what's the problem?' 'Er, well...' they said, 'he seems to have a candle stuck in his bottom.'

Ah.

Everyone has heard the stories about patients presenting to hospital with all manner of foreign bodies retained in their rectums. Anything from sex toys to shampoo bottles to light bulbs have had to be removed, even a whole frozen fish has been recorded. But this was the first (and last) time in my career that I had to actually deal with this particular problem.

'So', I asked the rather embarrassed young man before me, 'how did that get in there then?' His story was that the brothers of his ex-girlfriend had been so angry with him for breaking off their relationship, that they had attacked him and forcibly inserted said candle as a punishment. I didn't like to ask, but it was clear that he had sustained no other injuries at all.

I did rather think that if someone was declaring an interest in putting a 9 inch candle into my backside, I would have at least tried to resist and would certainly have had some evidence of defensive injuries about my person.

But still, it is not our place to question the patient too much and it still needed to be removed, regardless of the willingness with which it had been inserted. It was clear from the x-ray that it was wick down, so to speak, and therein lay the hope that it might be retrievable using some form of grabber. I decided that if I could at least get to see the wick, I ought to be able to get a hold of it and pull it out.

I asked the anaesthetist to administer some sedation to relax both the patient and his sphincter, and I inserted a sigmoidoscope (tool for inspecting the lower colon). After a certain degree of manoeuvring, I eventually managed to glimpse a bit of wick and quickly grabbed at it with a biopsy forceps. I had not realised that the forceps tip was pretty sharp and unfortunately it cut right through the wick. Now we were in trouble. There only remained about 3mm of wick protruding from the candle.

Don't forget this was central Belize, not a fully equipped NHS hospital, and there was a limited choice of instruments. Fortunately with a degree of pressure from above, through the abdomen, a little more sedation and the benefit of my long slim fingers, I was eventually able to grab the stump of wick with my fingertips and got the damned thing out.

I thought I deserved a decent thank you to be honest, but the moment the sedation had worn off, the patient made himself scarce without a word.

And he never calls or writes.

Gabriel Grüner

We weren't able to save this patient, but God knows we tried.

Gabriel Grüner was a senior correspondent with Stern magazine from Germany. He was covering the unrest in Kosovo and the rioting that spilled over into neighbouring Macedonia in the June of 1999.

He and his cameraman were caught up in the melee and shots were fired. An AK47 round entered the left side of his abdomen and exited through his upper back on the right side, just below the ribcage.

We were set up in a prefabricated shelter on an industrial compound on the outskirts of Skopje, the capital of Macedonia. This was a temporary stop in preparation for the planned helicopter insertion into Kosovo to provide surgical support for the UK Airborne Brigade that was tasked with stabilising Pristina once the Serb Army had withdrawn.

The facility consisted of one operating table, an air-mobile and versatile field operating table designed by Lt Col Frank MacVicar some thirty years before, and ten beds with appropriate numbers of Combat Medical Technicians (CMTs) and nursing personnel. We were equipped with basic surgical instruments, in order to provide life and limb-saving surgery, and a refrigerator containing 10 units of O negative donated blood.

Gabriel was brought to us by wheeled ambulance, arriving about 45 minutes after sustaining his injury. He was already profoundly shocked and needed immediate surgery. Blood was administered and we opened his abdomen through a long midline incision. For this operation I was the assistant, my general surgery colleague Barrie Price being the operating surgeon. Although I had covered general surgery as a junior, this was not a case for the inexperienced and I was more than happy to have a subsidiary role.

The track of the bullet was across the retroperitoneum, which means the back wall of the abdomen. This is where all the major vessels lie and is definitely 'tiger country', as well as being physically difficult to access, there being seemingly never-ending coils of intestine lying in the front, always managing to slip back into the way of desperate hands trying to find the source of haemorrhage.

The problem was the liver. It seemed like the main bleeding was from behind it and we just couldn't get there. 'I need an aortic clamp,' called Barrie, who was hoping that by temporarily stopping the flow of blood into the abdomen, we might stand a chance of identifying the bleeding vessels and controlling them.

No aortic clamp on the set, or in any set we had. 'You'll have to be the clamp,' said Barrie to me, 'use your thumb and index finger'. I pressed on the descending aorta as instructed, thereby tying up 50% of my assisting capacity, for what seemed like hours. It was in fact for about 45 minutes, but I eventually lost all feeling in those fingers, such was the pressure needed.

Despite all Barrie's experience and skill we just couldn't get to the damaged vessels. Despite using all the banked blood and the CMT's donating their own blood 'on the hoof', and despite all the anaesthetic tricks our colleague Malcolm Jowitt could think of, we lost the battle and Gabriel died on the table after approximately 3 hours of surgery.

It felt like the end of the world. It always does if you lose a patient, however it happens. The place was a wreck, the floor covered in blood, empty containers and swab packets. People stood around and just stared into the distance for a while, and no-one wanted to talk. We were done in.

The declared intention of the planners, sitting in their offices in London or elsewhere is that a two surgeon operating team deployed in isolation, will be able to undertake up to four major operations sequentially, if required. We had done one, and I rather doubt we would have been good for another for at least two hours. Maybe, if there was another Priority One casualty waiting, things would have been different but it's hard to imagine either of us would have been much use for a while.

Gabriel was taken away and transported back to Hamburg, his home town in Germany. When the next edition of Stern was published, his life and career were described in an editorial. Included in this was the report of the chief forensic pathologist in Hamburg, who had conducted the post mortem examination. He stated unequivocally that despite the efforts of the British operating team in Skopje, the injuries Gabriel had sustained were, in his opinion, unsurvivable.

Which was of some comfort at least.

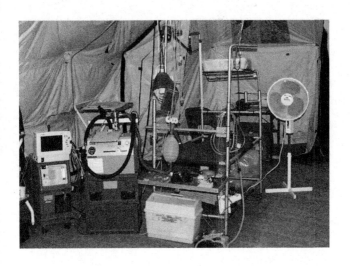

MacVicar operating table and anaesthetic machine

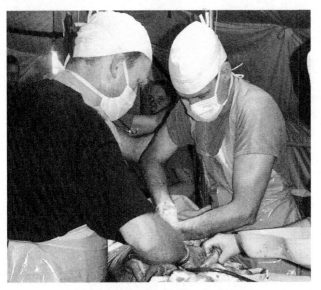

Barrie and Jonathan in deep

One for the high jump

This story is a sad one and for reasons that will become clear I cannot ask the patient for their permission. I will therefore change names etc but the details are absolutely true.

Jane was unhappy, really unhappy, and as a result she decided the only way out was to jump off the top floor of a multi-storey car park not far from the hospital. It was subsequently calculated that she would have fallen approximately 110 ft down onto the pavement.

Jane had never done parachute training or been taught how to fall as a stuntwoman. Despite that, she somehow managed to perform a pretty good demonstration of how to land from height, contacting with both feet flat on the ground, feet and knees together. It is unlikely that she was then able to roll as per the instruction manual, but she did avoid injuring her head which is pretty remarkable. There is good evidence from the scene that her Glasgow Coma Score was 15/15, indicating she was fully conscious throughout, more than can be said for a passer-by who fainted from the shock of witnessing a fully-grown female land from nowhere on the pavement, two feet away from him.

Jane was rushed to A&E and resuscitated promptly. There is a saying in the parachuting world if you come in backwards. It goes Heels, Harse, Head, Hospital. Jane avoided the head part but got everything else in between.

The recognised pattern of injuries caused by a fall from height includes fractures of the heel bone (os calcis), just below the knee (tibial plateau), hip joint, pelvis, sacrum, lumbar vertebrae and shoulder (from falling sideways after landing). Or all of the above. On both sides. In addition, there is a risk of rupture of either the liver or spleen inside the abdomen.

Jane broke all her bones as listed, but managed to avoid doing anything inside her abdomen or chest and thus was remarkably stable throughout her period of resuscitation. She required some urgent surgery though to stabilise her fractures and prevent them bleeding if possible. Broken bones bleed a great deal and the key thing is to keep them still if possible, and at the same time try and find a way to keep the joints moving. The best way in the emergency situation is to stabilise long bones and the pelvis with an external frame. Pins are placed via keyhole incisions into intact bone on either side of the fracture and then these pins are bolted to stabilising bars that span the fracture. That way a scaffold is built up around the affected limb, or across the front of the pelvis if that is fractured.

This process is necessarily different for every fracture and every patient and most trauma orthopaedic surgeons rather enjoy making it up as they go along, slowly creating a stable construct to hold the patient together. If possible one tries to avoid spanning across a joint such as the knee, so that early movement can be started in the days following the initial surgery. It is better for the joint, and ultimately the patient, if some movement can occur. This reduces swelling and pain and improves the chances of a good long-term outcome.

Jane looked like a half-built building after that first session in theatre but the fractures stopped bleeding quickly and she stabilised nicely. Although you can treat fractures with external frames until they heal, it is usually better to fix fractures with internal plates and screws if you can. It is quite important to get this done fairly quickly as, if you leave external pins in bone for more than a couple of weeks, the bone can get infected which is difficult to treat. And you would not want an internal plate to become infected as it may have to be removed to get the infection sorted.

Jane became the whole department's project for some months. We are a big group of specialists and we all do our own part. We have foot and ankle surgeons, knee and hip surgeons and spinal and shoulder experts. Everyone tries to stick to what they do best, except in the emergency situation, and that way the patient gets the best we can collectively offer.

Jane needed something from most of us and underwent many semi-elective operations to internally fix most of her fractures. As soon as she had recovered from one, she was listed for the next and she soon became used to these repeated interventions. It took time and must have been painful and seemingly never-ending for her but the plan worked and after about three months we were all delighted to see her up and mobilising on the ward with the physios.

Of course there was the issue of her mental state to contend with. She had absolutely meant to take her own life that day on the car park roof and it was no 'cry for help.' Through amazing good luck and her uncannily good landing technique, she had miraculously survived to tell the tale but were the same demons that drove her literally to the edge, still there waiting to re-emerge?

To be honest, I have no idea. I am an orthopaedic surgeon and I fix broken bones. Other doctors specialise in mental health and, together with psychologists and therapists, try to fix broken minds. I am sure that many of these specialists worked with Jane throughout her hospital stay and she certainly seemed to be getting happier on the surface, at least whenever I spoke to her.

Finally after 9 months or so she was ready for discharge. Plans would have been carefully made and one day she went home. There was no great fanfare to see her off as by then we had all moved on to dealing with lots of fresh cases on a daily basis. But it was good to know that collectively we had managed to put her back together.

Jane came back to A&E a couple of days later. Properly dead. When they removed her clothes, she was covered in what looked like plasters. In fact, it turned out they were Fentanyl patches. Fentanyl is a long acting opiate painkiller and she had been treated in hospital with these patches to control her pain from the injuries and all the operations. What no-one could have known was that she was secretly peeling them off and keeping them hidden in her locker. When she got home, she had a few drinks to relax her, and started to stick the patches on her arms and anywhere else she could. Eventually they made her fall asleep and she slowly slipped away.

Which has got to be easier than jumping off a car park.

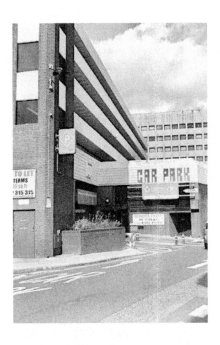

Victoria Road car park, Aldershot

The importance of AIRWAY

The supreme position of the airway in the hierarchy of resuscitation is drummed into every first-aider, paramedic, nurse, doctor and followers of Casualty and ER. 'A' comes before 'B' and so on. We are warned that to ignore the airway is a potential disaster and after 4 minutes with no viable airway, the patient's brain will be reduced to a sloppy bucket of dead neurones.

Maria was 31 and came from the Falls Road in Belfast. That almost certainly meant she was a staunch Roman Catholic with family or social links to the Provisional IRA. Or at least that is what we would have thought back in the mid 1980's when I happened to be involved in her care. I have no idea whether any of that was really true, except the fact that she did come from the Falls.

I was a Senior House Officer, which is one rank up from the bottom of the medical tree, when one is too inexperienced to be able to do anything very exciting, and senior enough to be blamed if anything goes wrong. I was on call for the burns unit in south east London one night when Maria was brought in. She had been involved in a house fire and had serious but not life-threatening burns to approximately 20% of her body area.

She had superficial burns around her face and neck and more serious full thickness, or 3rd degree, burns on her arms and chest. She was thought to have inhaled a small amount of smoke but was not considered to have significant inhalation injury as she could breathe and speak normally. Her burns were dressed with flamazine which is soothing and helps prevent infection, and she was given intravenous fluids to correct for fluid loss through the burns.

When I crawled back into bed at 2am, my wife, who was a burns-trained nurse, half woke up and told me that she could tell we had had a bad burn that night because she could smell it on my hands. Good to know.

The following day, tired as always, I struggled through a general surgical operating list, assisting in some major bowel operation I expect, and was finally released to go home at around 5pm. I thought I would swing by the burns unit on my way out of the hospital just to see how Maria was doing. Before I got to the main entrance, a nurse came rushing out of the door and said 'Oh, good you're here, come quickly!' Having no idea what the problem was I followed her in. It was clear that Maria was in real trouble. Her face had swollen up like a balloon and her mouth was a tiny shrunken hole surrounded by thick swollen lips. She was rasping and wheezing and desperately trying to get air into her lungs, writhing around in an attempt to find a position in which she could actually breathe. In short she was at the point of total respiratory arrest due to airway obstruction. Somehow this had slowly developed over the day without anyone realising, and she was now in dire straights.

AIRWAY my brain screamed at me. Normally one would pass a tube through the mouth into the trachea but not in Maria's case, as her mouth was too constricted. Same for her nose. The only way to save her was going to be a tracheostomy, which means cutting a hole in the front of the neck to open the trachea below the vocal cords. Everyone has heard the tale of some hero that performed a tracheostomy in the street using a pen-knife and a Bic biro tube. Unfortunately that is not real life, and I was no hero. And I had never so much as seen an actual tracheostomy, never mind done one. Gulp.

I called for a minor surgical kit and asked the nurses to get Maria lying flat on the bed. No time for local anaesthetic I'm afraid so sorry dear, this may sting a little. The problem with burns is that they cause a good deal of soft tissue swelling and I realised that I could not actually see or feel any recognisable anatomy on her neck. I knew the trachea was in the middle and that the carotids and jugulars were either side and that was about it.

Oh well. Be bold, I told myself, and I made a deep vertical incision right down into the trachea. I knew I had hit the spot as there was a huge rush of air as the poor patient took a massive breath in and filled her lungs. This was immediately matched by a tidal wave of venous bleeding from an unknown blood vessel that had also been cut. We managed to pass a small tube into the trachea to protect the airway and, by turning her head to the side, stopped her lungs from filling up with blood, but the bleeding just wouldn't stop despite pressure.

So, I realised, B (bleeding) really does come after A (airway), just like it says in all the books. Good to know. Trouble is I had now reached the limit of my capabilities and I had no idea what to do next. Fortunately medicine is a team sport and at this point help arrived in the form of a Senior Registrar who we will call Barrie. SRs are at the very top of the tree of training and in those days they had seen and done it all to the point of boredom while waiting for a consultant job to become available.

'Right' said Barrie, 'it looks like you may have pranged the anterior jugular'. This is a small insignificant vein that crosses the front of the neck and in Maria's case would have been engorged by her efforts to breathe against resistance.

'We'll just pop into theatre to sort that out. May have to split the sternum to get to it, but that's no bother,' said Barrie, duly managing to sound just a little bored. 'You get off home, you've done your bit,' he told me. So I did. Shaking like a leaf, I told my wife that I had almost certainly killed Maria and that when her Provo relatives found out where I lived, my knee-caps would be the least of my problems. Not a good feeling.

About an hour later Barrie called to say it was all sorted and that it just needed one suture to stop the bleeding. Maria was stable and not dead.

'Oh by the way, you saved her life, well done.'

Good to know.

Drilling for...oil?

Try and imagine the scene. We had just arrived at our new camp. I say camp, but I actually mean our designated patch of desert about 10 miles north of Kuwait City.

The date is the 28th February 1991, and we had been on the go for the best part of four days with perhaps a total of 6 hours sleep. We were Forward Surgical Team Alpha (FST A), attached to 7 Armoured Brigade's 1 Armoured Field Ambulance. In simple terms we were the surgical support for our half of the British troops that were involved in the push into Kuwait to kick out Saddam Hussein's army of occupation. FST B were looking after the other half of the Division.

Our war had started on the 24th with a move up to the Saudi border with Iraq, and the following day we crossed over in the wake of the Americans. There followed a mad cross-country dash as the Allied forces swept in from the west to overwhelm and rout the Iraqi Republican Guard. There was a slightly awkward moment on the second night when we managed to actually get in front of our own tanks, such was the enthusiasm of our Commanding Officer. Fortunately the Life Guards' Scimitar tanks that had been sent to destroy the rogue Iraqi column that we were thought to be, recognised our red crosses and didn't actually kill us. Thank you Major James Hewitt (*the* James Hewitt by the way).

At intervals along the journey we would be ordered to halt, set up a makeshift tented medical facility and treat casualties. The vast majority of these were Iraqi troops and what a bedraggled and weary lot they turned out to be. Most had, very sensibly, surrendered immediately when they saw our tanks approaching but a few were caught in the crossfire inevitably. We did have a few British casualties to deal with, mainly injured by US airplanes firing on them in error, the so-called blue-on-blue incidents. The most infamous of these was a pair of British Warrior armoured vehicles that were attacked by A10 Thunderbolt aircraft. We took several of the casualties from that encounter and boy were they cross.

Fortunately none were critical and I would expect the ones we treated would have made a full recovery. By the time we arrived at our patch of desert outside Kuwait City, we were totally exhausted, along with the whole Division. Never mind the armchair pundits saying we should have gone on to take Baghdad, we were in no shape to carry on without at least a couple of days' sleep. The tanks might have still been battle-worthy but the crews and the rest of us certainly weren't.

Anyway, despite the fatigue we still tried to manage whatever casualties found their way to our facility. That morning of the 28th turned out to be marred by a sandstorm, and the helicopters were unable to fly for a few hours. We had received an Iraqi casualty mid-morning who had sustained a bad head injury. This was not a bullet or fragment wound but a blunt injury from a fall or some other hard blow to the side of his head. He was deeply unconscious and we noted that his right pupil was fixed and dilated.

I don't know his name but let's call him Ali. Ali was in a bad way and, even without a scan, it seemed pretty clear that he had bleeding inside his skull causing the right pupil to be fixed. It was a classic extra-dural haematoma and without treatment it was likely he would die as his brain tried to slowly squeeze its way out of the hole in the base of his skull. What Ali needed was someone to drill a hole into his skull to let the pressure off. This is following exactly the same principle as when you have a haematoma under your finger-nail and you release it by pushing a hot paperclip through the nail.

If the helicopters had been flying, we would have sent him back to the field hospital in Saudi where they would have had much better facilities to operate. We had no more than a stretcher on the sand and some very basic instruments. But we *did* have a brace and bit, thoughtfully included in the surgical kit we had acquired (stolen) in Saudi before we moved out to the desert. Normally one would use a power drill to make a hole in the skull but that wasn't an option here; it was back to basics and a good old fashioned hand drill for Ali's craniotomy.

Now this operation I had at least seen, if not actually done. In surgery the saying is 'see one, do one, teach one'; if you are very unlucky the fourth is 'have one'. I decided to skip the second and, as my combat medical technician Cpl Smith was keen as mustard and perfectly well skilled, he did the actual drilling, something he was unlikely to ever get another chance to do.

Bone is hard and you have to push. Ever so slowly the hole deepened and suddenly we were rewarded with a spurt of dark red blood, so dark it actually looked like oil, which considering we were in Kuwait seemed quite appropriate. No anaesthetic was required of course as Ali was deeply unconscious but even after a few minutes he began to show signs of movement. After sucking as much old blood and clot out of the craniotomy as we could, the hole was left open and lightly packed with gauze.

And then we waited. After about 10 minutes Ali definitely started to make purposeful movements and miraculously his previously fixed and dilated pupil returned to normal size and reacted to light.

I can't tell you that he regained consciousness before he departed on a Royal Navy helicopter for a Red Cross hospital, but we were certainly hopeful. Sadly we never did find out what the eventual outcome was but I'd like to think we gave him a fighting chance.

I'd say that was rather better than drilling for oil, wouldn't you?

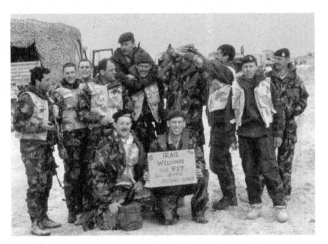

FST A at the Saudi-Iraq border 25 Feb 91

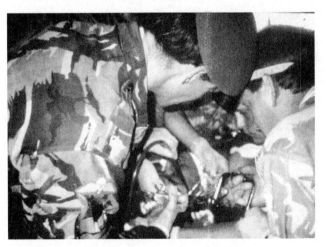

Drilling for extra-dural haematoma 28 Feb 91

A textbook case

This case really is 'textbook'. I say that because it formed the basis of a chapter I was asked to write for a textbook; the title of the chapter was 'Multiple Injuries' and that is exactly what this patient had.

It was a Range Rover versus a SmartCar. At an estimated combined speed of 70 mph. Head on. It is actually rather surprising that the SmartCar driver made it to hospital, but the paramedics did a great job and the journey time was short.

The patient was a 54 year old female in previously good health. The airbag had deployed and as a result she had no head injury. Initial investigations in the emergency department revealed multiple open fractures including both femurs, right patella, right tibia, left humerus and right os calcis (heel bone). There was an unstable fracture of the second cervical vertebra and a closed multi-level fracture of the left humerus.

As well as all the broken bones, this lady had also ruptured her liver which was bleeding inside the abdomen. Fortunately her pelvis was intact and as said, she had no sign of a head injury.

All this adds up to a set of life-threatening injuries with a very high expected mortality. Good effective resuscitation at the scene and in the ED meant that we, the surgeons, had a good chance of saving her - if we did the right things *at the right time*.

It is tempting to think that all these injuries should be treated as soon as possible and indeed in previous decades that is exactly what would have been attempted. It was not unusual to hear about 12 or 14 hour operations to deal with all the injuries on the first day. Most of these patients survived the operation to get to ITU, but sadly a significant proportion subsequently went downhill and died in the next few days or weeks. It became clear that the extended time in theatre on Day 1 seemed to be the cause of this.

Patients get cold very quickly after injury and lying naked on an operating table makes this even worse. Even if the temperature in theatre is kept high, uncomfortably so for the operators, the body temperature of the patient will rapidly fall. This is partly due to immobility and also open wounds are a major source of heat loss. What does a low temperature do?

Well, a major consequence is reduction in the ability for blood to clot and this then leads to more bleeding and more heat loss. It can be impossible to correct this with blood products, which may themselves be cold, and the situation spirals downwards. If the body is cold, the blood supply to major organs will start to reduce, and a prolonged period of poor blood supply to the kidneys, liver and heart can cause irreversible damage that manifests as failure of multiple organ systems a few days later.

The key principle nowadays is Damage Control. This means do the minimum to stabilise the situation and maximise the chances of the patient living to fight another day. Clearly, active bleeding must be stopped and in this case the liver laceration needed urgent attention. Bleeding from multiple fractures can be catastrophic and a quick way of stopping this is required, not a perfect and complex reconstruction of every fracture but a rapid 'first aid' type of fixation using either external bars or splints.

When multiple surgical teams are working together it also helps if someone is clearly in charge, and a rough plan of attack is agreed upon in advance. In this patient's case, that team leader was a very experienced anaesthetist who controlled who did what when, in a similar way to an orchestra conductor.

So what happened? She was in theatre within 2 hours of arrival at the hospital. Her neck was in a stiff collar which was sufficient to protect the cervical fracture. After she was anaesthetised, the general surgeons opened her abdomen and were able to pack the liver laceration and stop the bleeding.

While the abdomen was being dealt with, the legs were put in traction to keep them still and straight, again reducing bleeding significantly. Once the abdomen had been closed, the orthopods (orthopaedic surgeons) working as two teams then rapidly applied an external frame to each leg, with fixation pins above and below the fractures, on the right side including the knee joint so that the whole leg was fixed in one piece. Wounds were washed and packed but not sewn up. The left humerus was put into a plaster half-cast. And then we stopped.

2 hours max and we had the situation under control with a good blood pressure, no active bleeding and a near normal temperature. This lady was clearly going to need many more operations to definitively fix all the fractures, but these could wait for a few days or even weeks without compromising the outcome.

She remained stable on ITU overnight and I was amazed the next morning to find that she was sitting up, fully alert and eating breakfast!

I subsequently saw her some years later when she was in for a minor unrelated operation. She seemed pretty much normal apart from a slight limp.

You never forget a case like that.

Every cloud...

I was unable to contact this patient so I have changed her name for reasons you might appreciate later.

Lisa was a twenty-something single female who had annoying hip pain. It had started a year or so before I met her and had gradually become worse, and was starting to affect her everyday life. She had pain on exercise and after sitting or driving and she had noticed her hip was stiff and difficult to move fully. The pain was in her groin mainly and there was an annoying click in there when she moved in a certain way. She had a boyfriend and this hip pain was starting to spoil their intimate moments as well as restricting what they could get up to.

I met her for the first time in outpatients where she had been referred by her GP. I specialise in young adult hip problems and this sounded very much like she had a tear in the rim cartilage around the hip joint. This cartilage sometimes tears as the result of an injury, but more commonly it is damaged as a consequence of a condition called femoro-acetabular impingement. This is when the shape of the ball and the socket in the hip are not quite the same, and there is a mismatch leading to problems.

In simple terms, the ball is not perfectly spherical and is very slightly egg-shaped or ovoid. Over the years this causes high friction on the inside of the socket and eventually it starts to

cause symptoms. If it was a bearing in an engine, it woul
eventually wear out and break - the same happens in the hi
and the first sign of trouble is usually pain.

We confirmed the diagnosis with an MRI scan and this clear
showed that the head shape was wrong and the cartilage wa
torn. When this condition was first recognised, some twent
years ago, the treatment was to open the hip joint, dislocat
it and shave off the abnormal bone. This often worked but
was a pretty large hammer to crack a relatively small nut an
by 2010 most of us were gaining experience in doing thi
through keyhole surgery - hip arthroscopy - where a 4 mr
camera is passed into the joint and micro-instruments ar
used to deal with the problem.

I explained to Lisa that I thought this would be the bes
option for her and after some discussion she agreed to go o
the list. I would have warned her that there was a very lov
risk of infection after this operation as it is done though tin
incisions, but that the pulling and stretching necessary t
allow access to the hip might cause some temporar
numbness post op.

In fact, the operation is done with the patient in traction an
a good deal of force is needed to get the head to pull out o
the socket enough to allow the camera and instruments t
pass safely into the joint. It is no good just pulling on the le
though, and there has to be counter-traction to allow th
head to distract. This takes the form of a padded pos

positioned between the patient's legs, up against the pubic bone.

In male patients every care is taken to ensure that the testicles are out of the way as severe damage could be caused if one or both were squashed up against the post, whatever the padding used. In females, there is nothing to move out of the way but in my experience up to that point, the worst I had seen was a little numbness post op which always resolved quickly.

The operation proceeded uneventfully and was over and done with in under an hour. The time the traction was on was about 30 minutes, so not long really. Post op, Lisa seemed fine and the hip wasn't too painful so she went home that evening. Job done.

Four days later, when I was relaxing after dinner at home, I received a call from the on-call consultant in Obstetrics & Gynaecology. She had been called into A&E to see Lisa who had presented with severe bruising and trauma to her nether regions. This had started within a few hours of the operation and had become much worse over the next three days, to the point where she was really worried. The whole area was numb and pain wasn't a real issue for her.

I was told that the poor lady's clitoris was very swollen and bruised and my colleague was very worried that it may have been so badly damaged that it might need removal.

How awful. I had done this operation hundreds of times and never seen this complication before. There are cases of genital damage reported in the literature but usually these were as a result of very long traction times causing sustained pressure down below. In this case we had only used traction for thirty minutes and it seemed really unfair that this lady was in so much trouble.

The following morning I rushed in to see Lisa on the gynae ward and profusely apologised of course. She was remarkably sanguine I thought and, as she wasn't in that much discomfort, didn't appear to be too worried really. She was scheduled to go to theatre later in the morning to allow for a full inspection and any necessary tissue debridement.

I waited anxiously for my consultant colleague to call me after the operation, and was hugely relieved to hear that things were not as bad as had been feared. Nothing had needed to be removed and she thought that, given time, the area would settle down and heal.

Eight weeks later I saw that Lisa was on my clinic list for a follow-up appointment. With considerable trepidation I went out to the waiting area in outpatients to call her in. To my relief she stood up with a big smile on her face and walked briskly into my clinic room.

'Er, how's the hip?' I asked. 'Brilliant', she replied, 'All the pain has gone and I am starting to get back to the gym', she said.

I examined her hip and sure enough it moved freely without pain, and the three keyhole wounds had healed nicely. 'Um, and what about the other problem?' I asked nervously.

'What problem?', she replied with just the hint of a smile.

'Well, you know, the *bruising* that you had to come in with a few days later', I responded, not wishing to be too anatomical. As orthopods, we don't generally find it necessary, or particularly easy, to discuss patients' genitalia as a routine.

"Oh that', she said, 'It's fine, thank you'.

What a relief. I could, and perhaps should, have left it at that I suppose. She said it was fine, so I guess it *was* fine. But still...

'Er, great, so it's all settled down and back to normal then?' I asked.

'Oh yes', she said.

'Um, so all the bruising has gone then?' I asked.

'Yes thank you', she replied and I am sure there was a twinkle in her eye.

'…and the numbness?' I enquired.

'Oh, yes that's all gone' she answered. 'In fact, it's actually rather *more* sensitive down there now than it was before '. And this time she was definitely smiling.

'Thank you', I said.

'No, no, thank *you*', she replied, and off she went with a spring in her step.

Guns and alcohol don't mix

Bosnia, June 1998.

The Balkans had been simmering since the early 90s and in central Bosnia-Herzegovina there existed reasonably peaceful co-existence of the warring parties by 1998. The United Nations had established a peacekeeping force throughout the former Yugoslavia, to which the UK contributed forces and therefore medical support.

For army surgeons, the four week tours of duty in the village of Sipovo in central Bosnia were regarded as a break from the routine of NHS hospital life and a chance to relax, sleep a little, take some exercise and maybe even write up that overdue research paper. The medical facility, 'hospital', was sited in a disused warehouse into which shipping so-containers had been placed to provide treatment areas and living accommodation. Although fairly rudimentary, it was warm and dry and cleaner than many places we had been asked to work in over the years.

The operating 'theatre' was in one such container, and although a bit cramped if you were over 5'10'' tall, it could take an operating table and anaesthetic machine and there was enough space to make surgery possible, if not as comfortable as in a full-sized theatre back home. There were no cats to swing so the fact that one couldn't was not a problem, and being military we were used to adapting and making the best of what we were given.

Not that there was much in the way of surgery to be getting to grips with. Plenty of surgeons would pass their four weeks without doing so much as an in-growing toenail. The occasional abscess would need lancing and there would be training injuries to manage, but there was nothing too dramatic to do for most of us.

So, when a local Bosnian farmer was brought in one evening with his foot half hanging off, there was considerable excitement all round. He had been at the Slivovitz (Šljivovica in Serbian), which is a damson plum based locally distilled fire-water of 80-90% proof. They all seemed to drink it in vast quantities and most appeared to thrive on it.

Our man Teufik was about 60 and he had been out patrolling his land, armed with a single-barrelled shotgun of questionable age. Judging by his demeanour, it is likely that he had been drinking plenty of Slivo to help pass the time and may just have had one too many. He had attempted to climb over a stile and had slipped. The loaded shotgun had accidentally discharged at this point and, as it was pressing against his left foot at the time, caused a pretty dramatic injury.

Someone had thoughtfully applied a tourniquet to stop most of the bleeding but it was clear there was no way we were going to be able to save his foot. The local interpreter was a nice enough lad but when I asked him to explain to Teufik that we were going to have to amputate the leg just below the knee, he became quite upset and refused to. Try as I might, I couldn't get him to explain to the patient what we needed to do. In the end, I had to resort to sign language and make sawing motions with my hand at the level of Teufik's upper calf, to get my message across. This was accompanied by much nodding, smiling and a questioning thumbs-up gesture on my part and eventually it dawned on Teufik that he was going to lose part of his leg.

Now, the principle of 'informed consent' is considered hugely important in modern surgery. It is essential that the patient should have a clear understanding of the options open to them, the exact nature of the proposed treatment and be fully aware of all possible complications. In addition, they should be given the opportunity to reflect and to not be rushed into making a decision about whether to proceed. Hmm.

We had no option under the circumstances on that day in that place, but to accept Teufik's eventual and somewhat reluctant thumbs-ups gesture as the only 'informed consent' we were going to get, and we whisked him into the operating theatre without further delay.

It was not a difficult amputation and it was completed without complication within an hour. The only slight moment of levity was when the clamp I had placed on the tibial artery slipped, and the Royal Engineer observer we had allowed in to watch the operation (and who was standing at the foot of the operating table) was hit full in the centre of his chest with a jet of arterial blood, causing him to collapse in a dead faint.

Well, it's not for everyone I suppose.

Never EVER treat family

My daughter, Charlie, mastered walking quite early and so by the time she was 19 months old she was looking for new challenges. As I had only recently completed parachute training and was still enthusiastic about it (having done very few jumps and never been injured), it was only natural that I should teach her the basic techniques. Surely that was reasonable?

Anyway, one Sunday afternoon in Woolwich we had a go and she was good. To start with. With me holding onto her hands she got the hang of jumping from the dining room table and was able to reliably land nicely with her feet and knees together. In fact she was so proficient that it quickly became obvious that my hands were unnecessary and she prepared for her first 'solo' jump.

'Red on, green on, go!' I shouted. She went. She fell. And she landed like a bag of potatoes, all that training and practice forgotten, feet miles apart. There was an ominous crack from somewhere close, followed by two full seconds of absolute silence... then all hell broke loose. Charlie screamed in pain, my wife screamed in anger (at me for some reason), and her younger brother Richard giggled uncontrollably.

'You idiot, you've broken her leg!' my wife shouted. Hardly fair, surely it was just bad technique, I thought, but obviously didn't say.

'She's just sprained her ankle', I did say, 'they always crack like that'. Oops.

Things calmed down a little and for a couple of hours Charlie seemed fine - sitting on the sofa. Weight-bearing was not so fine I'll admit and in fact she couldn't stand on that leg at all, so eventually I agreed we should probably take this further.

The nearest A&E was miles away and was bound to be crowded on a Sunday afternoon (really?), so I decided to pop across to the Queen Elizabeth Military Hospital where I was a Senior House Officer in general surgery at the time. It didn't have an A&E department but the on-call radiographer would no doubt be happy to do a quick x-ray to prove that nothing was broken. He was, and *it* was. She had a spiral fracture of the lower third of the tibia, undisplaced, but definitely there on the pictures.

The thing about that particular fracture pattern is that it is commonly seen in cases of Non-Accidental Injury, (aka child abuse).

No matter, I thought, both Charlie and I both knew this was *not* child abuse and she freely admitted she had messed up her landing. Well, sort of. What she needed now was a nice plaster cast, not a nice social worker, and I knew just the man for the job. The duty theatre tech was good at plasters, and without delay we had Charlie nicely encased in a POP (Plaster of Paris) from her toes to her bum. Job done.

Overnight I began to wonder how it might look to a dispassionate professional with an interest in child safeguarding. Probably not great I decided and never mind Charlie's broken tibia, I felt *I* needed some protection as well. First thing on Monday morning I sought out the senior orthopaedic surgeon, not only in the hospital but also in the Army, Brigadier Graham Stock, Consultant Adviser in Orthopaedics. I explained the whole situation and gave particular emphasis to the quality of instruction given, and the disappointing performance by my 19 month old daughter leading to this unfortunate training accident.

'You bloody idiot,' was his professional opinion, and I could see my aspirations to become an orthopod leaving the building. 'You should know she doesn't need a full leg cast for that fracture, 'Get her into a below-knee right away, or her knee will get stiff'. Right, sorry Sir, my mistake. Phew.

Charlie loved her cast and after four weeks it had been colourfully decorated and she was sorry to have to have it removed. Other than being inexplicably hairy for several years, her leg recovered very quickly and she had no further trouble. Although she never showed much interest in parachuting after that.

A month or two later, I was busy on the wards when a call come through for me. 'It's Sam Baker', the voice said. 'I'm a social worker with the Woolwich Child Protection team, and I gather your daughter was injured at home recently and doesn't appear to have been treated in the usual way...' It took me a few awful minutes to realise it was the disguised voice of my House Officer, finally given away by the uncontrolled giggling on the end of the line.

He's a GP now, as despite showing early promise, his career in hospital medicine never really took off for some reason.

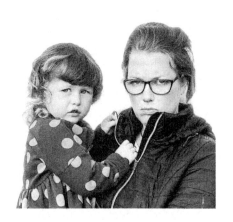

Surely she's not still cross with me?
(Charlie pictured with her daughter, my equally disgusted granddaughter, Livvy).

The Queen's English

I spent 12 months on Fellowship in Baltimore, Maryland in 1992-93. Being a Brit in the US was generally quite agreeable as they seem to like us for whatever reason. I found that the British accent went down a storm and I was often told it made me sound like David Niven or James Bond. In fact, I realised that if you kept a straight face you could get away with almost anything if you spoke the Queen's.

The hospital I worked in - Shock Trauma - was a trauma unit and did nothing else but. It took the most severely injured patients from around the city and the state, and there was no A&E - you either arrived by ambulance or helicopter, and there were no walk-ins. This tended to mean that the cases were complex and interesting, in contrast to a British A&E department where a large proportion of the attendees really should have gone to see their GP instead.

The Americans do trauma really well. They have State-wide systems with good coordination between first responders and hospitals. In Maryland this was a refined setup and the central hub was the R Adams Cowley Shock Trauma Centre, located in West Baltimore on the edge of the 'bad lands' into which I was firmly advised not to venture, especially at night.

Cowley was a visionary in the 1960's and he developed Maryland's model which has subsequently been widely copied. He recognised that trauma victims did better if they were treated in dedicated facilities set apart from a general hospital. Rapid transfer from the scene of the injury, by helicopter if possible, early resuscitation and/or surgery and specialised rehabilitation leads to improved outcomes for patients. It is a simple, but expensive, concept.

We ran teams and often there would be several major cases going on simultaneously as the numbers would sometimes demand that. The hospital had 6 operating theatres, all of which could be used at once. On one particular Saturday in November, Fox News sent in a team of reporters and cameramen to give a snapshot of life in a trauma unit for a documentary. This kind of reality TV was already popular in the US, as it is now in the UK.

As it was busy and as I was becoming a little more competent by this stage, I was allowed to undertake an operation on my own while the consultants and other residents were busy elsewhere in the department. My case was a 'Ped struck' which is short for 'Pedestrian struck by vehicle'. He was a well-to-do 35 year old man who had wandered into the path of a large American sedan and had suffered open fractures of both his legs below the knee. Both tibias were broken but he had no other injuries of note and was conscious and stable on arrival.

Unlike many of the clientele we treated, this man was prosperous and successful in his work. I forget exactly but he was probably in insurance or finance or something similar, certainly not a typical trauma victim, who tended to be from the rougher side of the street. He had been out drinking with friends and had had one too many before stepping off the kerb, hence his accident. He loved the fact that his surgeon was a Brit and like all Americans assumed that we all know each other in England, so did I know his friend from London and had I met the Queen, etc.

I assured him I had never had tea at Buckingham Palace and explained that I needed to fix both his broken legs with a long rod inside the bone called an intramedullary nail. Each side would take an hour or so and with luck, he should be up and walking within a few days.

We proceeded to the Operating Room (they don't call them theatres in the States), and I duly went about my business. When you deal with just one broken tibia, you can judge the correct position to fix it, especially the rotation, by comparing it with the other - intact - side. Some people's feet point forwards, some splay out a little but usually that is by no more than 15 or so degrees. It is polite to try and give the patient a 'matching pair' so that they look normal afterwards.

Unfortunately, his fractures were quite complex and it was impossible to put the bones together precisely. The long nail went in easily enough on the first side, and held the fracture still, but I then needed to pass screws across the bone and through the nail, both above and below the fracture to fix the rotation and the length. Judging the position of the foot relative to the rest of the leg is done with what is known as the 'mark-one eyeball', and you have to make a call on what looks right as there is no gauge to tell you. One does one's best, but human error does come into play at times.

In other words, I may not have got it *exactly* right.

And, there was no normal side to compare it with as that was still broken awaiting repairs. Still, it looked good enough and I was pleased overall with the way that side went. Maybe it was just a *tad* over-rotated and perhaps the foot pointed out a *tiny* bit more than I had planned for?

We moved on. The second side was technically easier (you always do the worst side first in case there is a power cut or some other disaster). That was a much simpler fracture and the fixation was straightforward. When it came to deciding on the rotation of the foot, at least I now had something to compare it with, the first side. I duly used the eyeball trick and stood back to assess my work. Hmm, that margin of error thing again, but overall they looked pretty similar from the foot of the table and I was happy enough. Job done. His wounds healed up nicely and he was up walking three days later, ready to go home soon after that.

Remember that Fox News team I mentioned? They had not been in my operating room as there was probably something more exciting and juicy going on elsewhere in the hospital at the time, so I had not had the pressure of being live on TV while doing my operation.

But, they came back after three months to do a follow-up and unbeknown to me, my 'ped struck' patient had used his influence to persuade the producer to interview him live on the programme, and to surprise me by publicly thanking me for saving his legs.

It was classic live TV. Unsuspecting doctor ambushed by reporter and cameraman. Hideously grateful patient pumping my hand in the glare of the TV lights. Me stuttering something banal about 'just doing my job' etc. Patient walking off down the corridor, long lingering view from behind…

…whilst doing his best Charlie Chaplin impression with his feet pointing at ten-to-two at best. And with my name scrolling across the bottom of the screen.

I was so glad it was only shown in America, but like I said, you can get away with almost anything if you speak the Queen's.

The kids from Kosovo

Content warning: This story contains distressing situations and events and is intended for an adult audience only.

My last operational tour before leaving the Army was in Kosovo in 1999. After years of the Balkans being embroiled in various conflicts, Croatia, Bosnia, Serbia all at each other's throats, the last region to settle was Kosovo. NATO had needed to get involved and, after a bombing campaign by the US and UK, the Serbs were persuaded to leave the country for good.

This left a vacuum that was initially filled by Russia and, to prevent them taking control, 5 Airborne Brigade were quickly flown into Pristina to restore order. There is impressive TV footage of the robust Brigadier Adrian Freer, Commander 5 AB Bde, facing down his Russian equivalent at the gates of Pristina airport - and winning the battle of wills.

A single light surgical team was deployed to support British operations and we based ourselves in a disused factory in the suburbs of the city. We consisted of two surgeons - one general surgeon, one orthopod (me) - two anaesthetists, four operating department technicians and enough nurses to staff ten beds. Not exactly a hospital but we had had worse and knew how to make it work. We were used to treating soldiers and they don't need all the frills.

Although our mission was to provide support for UK troops, inevitably we became involved in treating locals, and with no functioning hospital in the city, we soon started getting civilians   dropping in and also being brought to us by ambulance or private car.

There were many we could not help and the majority really just needed to see a GP. However, it soon became apparent that some of the Serb soldiers who by now had vanished back to Serbia, had left little souvenirs behind in the Kosovan houses they had commandeered.

By which I mean booby traps.   Packets of explosive mixed with nuts and bolts, strategically placed on the tops of doors so that they went off when the door was opened. We had a few patients that had returned home from exile in Albania, only to find they had been left just such a house-warming present.

Whereas one is conditioned to soldiers being violent towards each other, after all it's what they're trained for, there is something really rather nasty about getting at civilians in this way, and the Balkans was particularly notorious for this kind of ethnic persecution. There are all manner of horror stories from this awful decade in the former Yugoslavia and we were fortunate to only have to witness the very end of it.

The subjects of this particular chapter were four children, all brothers and sisters, who were brought into our facility one day. The interpreter explained that they were orphans and that they had witnessed their father being shot after he, and they, had been made to watch their mother being gang-raped by drunken Serb soldiers. As if this wasn't horrific enough, they had then been told to run away and the soldiers took pot shots at them with AK47s to see who could hit them from the greatest range. What fun.

Fortunately the soldiers were too drunk to aim accurately and as a result none of the children had been fatally injured. All four had limb wounds, by then a couple of weeks old. They were undernourished and pale and the resigned and flat look in their eyes and their totally defeated demeanour is something that I will never forget. We patched them up, splinted their fractures which fortunately did not seem to be infected, gave antibiotics and vitamins, and passed them on to the International Committee of the Red Cross downtown.

When I returned home after my tour of duty, I found that I would be playing in the garden with my own four children and would suddenly and vividly get a flash-back to those kids in Kosovo. It might last for several minutes, during which I could do nothing but stand and stare into the distance with tears in my eyes.

Being a senior doctor and a para, I did not of course recognise that I had Post Traumatic Stress Disorder, or at least a mild version of it. On the day I subsequently gave a presentation on our Kosovo tour to the hospital staff at lunchtime, and broke down in tears in front of all my colleagues, the penny finally dropped.

And sure enough, talking about it was all I needed to do.

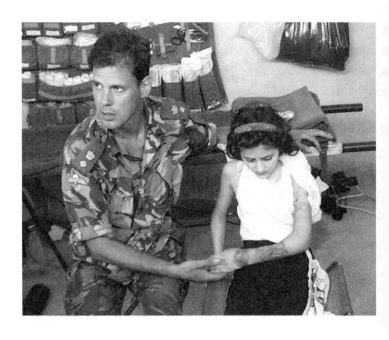

One of the Kosovan children. My face says it all

Mad cows

This story is about two people. They were a nice middle-aged, middle-class married couple who went for a nice walk in the middle of a field in the middle of a warm summer's evening.

When some time later they were lying in the A&E Department of my hospital, I was telephoned by the registrar on call for orthopaedics to tell me that these nice people wished to use their private medical insurance to fund their on-going treatment in the private ward of the hospital.

When I told him that I didn't generally take private trauma cases, he struggled not to laugh and said that regardless of that, I really ought to come and see them anyway as it would definitely make my evening. He wouldn't divulge any further details but knowing him to have a good sense of humour, I decided to pop in and see what could be causing so much interest.

I was not disappointed. James and Jennifer had indeed been out for a nice country walk that evening, and had followed the public footpath signs into and across a large sloping grassy field. At the far end of the field there was a medium-sized herd of Friesian cows, maybe 15 to 20 in number. The cows were minding their own business and appeared to be no threat. As James and Jennifer did not have a dog, they could see no reason not to proceed on with their walk, anticipating that the cows would quietly move away as they approached.

As they drew nearer, one of the cows looked up, noticed the walkers and moo'd loudly. Immediately the other cows joined in with the moo'ing, or rather bellowing, and turned to stare hard at our couple. Then, instead of moving off, they started to walk quite purposely towards them. This was so surprising that James and Jennifer didn't think to turn and run but stood patiently waiting, assuming quite reasonably that the cows would stop and back off. After all that's what cows do isn't it?

This particular herd appeared not to have read the rule book and instead of 'cowing' away, they advanced rapidly and before they knew it our walkers were surrounded by what were seemingly very angry beasts. They were jostled and nudged and pushed by big wet smelly noses and it was as if the cows were actually trying to crush them with their bodies.

And then they both slipped on the wet and muddy ground which is when it became really frightening. They found themselves literally under the hooves of these massive beasts and could not get away. They were trampled on by several large feet and both sustained significant fractures and one dislocated knee joint. They were screaming out in fear and pain and then...

…the madness passed and all of a sudden the cows went all quiet and calm again. They moved away from the injured couple and drifted off back to their corner of the field without so much as a backward glance. As if it had never happened.

James and Jennifer were in trouble. They were both in agony and neither could begin to walk or even crawl. They shouted for help and then they carried on screaming for someone, anyone, to come to their aid. After about ten long minutes another walker heard them and hurried over. He at least had a mobile phone and was able to call 999. At last an ambulance arrived but unfortunately wasn't able to negotiate the field to collect the patients.

The other person to turn up at this point was the farmer who owned both the field and the cows. One imagines he would have been very embarrassed to find that the cows he had put in a field which was crossed by a public footpath had in fact attacked and badly injured a pair of innocent walkers.

One would have thought. Apparently he was not so much embarrassed as furious, and voiced his opinion that the walkers must have done something to provoke his normally placid and peaceful beasts of burden. In the end after much grumbling he brought his tractor and trailer to the party and the pair were thus brought on a flatbed to the waiting ambulance. Not exactly the way they expected to end their evening stroll.

Back in A&E, I was of course the model of concern and courtesy. These nice people were intending to pay handsomely for their ongoing treatment and it would have been both rude and unproductive to allow so much as the hint of a smile to cross my face. Even the sight of smeared cow dung on Jennifer's Harris Tweed skirt produced not a single twinkle.

I went on to fix their bones and together with a colleague, reconstructed the dislocated knee. The national papers were full of the story and it seemed that there had been a previous issue with that particular group of cows. Surely they had not been trained to repel walkers who dared to use the footpath through their field?

Perish the thought.

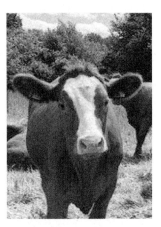

This is OUR field!

Frank
by
Hugh Chissell

Frank had been through a sudden and painful break up of his marriage and was left at home alone. He was clearly very upset and not thinking straight. He warned his neighbours that something big was going to happen at midnight.

And sure enough it did.

At five to midnight, he sawed through the main gas supply to his house in Southampton and at midnight he struck a match. The ensuing explosion blew the house apart. Frank was blown out of the house into the street in the moments before the house collapsed. He found himself alive with burns on his hands and face, but was otherwise apparently uninjured. The house was a pile of rubble and on fire.

The emergency services took Frank to the local A&E in Southampton and after assessing him they realised all he had was some flash burns and, amazingly, no other injuries. He was then transferred to the local burns unit arriving in the early hours of the morning.

Frank was clearly not in a good place mentally. Firstly he had tried to kill himself and secondly, he was very angry at his failure to achieve his primary aim. We tried to calm him down and dressed his burns with flamazine dressings. He seemed to settle down and I left him in the care of the nurses.

In these types of cases we always asked for a psychiatric opinion early on, as frequently these patients needed to be sectioned under the Mental Health Act. First thing the next morning, before going to participate in an operating list, I called the local psychiatric hospital and asked if someone would visit Frank on the burns unit.

The next thing I remember was being fast bleeped to the burns unit at the end of the morning to say that Frank had absconded.

I was unscrubbed and went down straightaway in my theatre greens and clogs. As I crossed the outdoor space between the hospital and the burns unit, the psychiatrist arrived in an ancient Mercedes accompanied by his spaniel.

It was one of those times when you meet someone who really does look like his dog. As he got out of his car I told him that Frank had left the premises - he replied with a glint in his eye, rubbing his hands together:

'Great, we can *definitely* section him now.'

The burns unit of the hospital, which was in a rural location at and the edge of the sprawling World War 2 ex-military hospital, overlooked green fields with a slope down to a small stream and a country lane leading to the pub where we used to have a swift drink after work.

I looked over to the field and saw Frank wearing his clothes and a duffle coat with bandages flying behind him, heading off at a rate of knots being chased by about half the nursing staff from the burns unit.
It looked like something out of the Benny Hill show. The psychiatrist plus spaniel and myself, still in theatre greens, followed in hot pursuit.

Cut off by the stream on a cold December day, even Frank wasn't mad enough to try and wade across. He headed along the side of the stream to another country lane and headed down this towards a T-junction. At this point three police cars arrived, one on each lane, and Frank was headed off, his brief bid for freedom curtailed by the long arm of the law.

We tried to persuade him to come quietly and after a short time he got into one of the police cars. Several cars drove past as we were doing this and pointed at us. I realised that the only person not wearing normal clothes in this group was myself, so obviously members of the public must have thought *I* was the escaped felon. Luckily the police arrested the correct person and Frank was taken to the local secure psychiatric unit.

The following week I visited Frank in the secure unit with my senior registrar. Apart from having difficulty identifying the staff from the patients, my main recollection is that Frank was housed in a cell with padding on the walls and that the only daylight was coming from a small window made of glass bricks near the ceiling.

He refused to have anything to do with treating his burns and every time they were dressed he ripped the bandages off within a few minutes. Amazingly, after a few more visits we discharged him as all his burns had healed without even a scar.

I've always wondered what happened to Frank.

Medice, cura te ipsum
(Physician heal thyself – Luke 4:23)

My most difficult patient was myself.

In 1996 I returned to 5 Airborne Brigade as a consultant surgeon, after a 6 year break for surgical training. If you go more than one year without parachuting, you have to complete a refresher course which consists of ground training, relearning how to fall and roll safely, and then complete three jumps in a single day at RAF Brize Norton.

Parachuting is *not* like riding a bike, and you do forget how to do it properly. If you actually listen to the instructors and concentrate on what you are doing during the ground training then I am sure the jumps are straightforward. If you don't, and you forget that in the 6 years you have been away they have introduced a new kind of parachute which has a faster forward speed than the old ones, you might land less than perfectly - just saying.

All three of my jumps that day were what are referred to as 'side rights', which means you land travelling from left to right and have to roll onto your right side after your feet hit the ground. If you are travelling rather faster than you should be at that point, you do land quite heavily on your right hip. If you do that three times in a day and the third time it *really* hurts, then it's not surprising that when you have driven 60 miles home in the evening, you can't actually get out of the car without help.

As a new consultant in my hospital and as a Major in my parachute unit, I did not feel inclined to make much of my 'bruised' hip and after a couple of weeks people stopped asking why I was limping. Slowly the pain went away, and as we were always taught in the Brigade, pain is just weakness leaving the body, so I was eventually 'good to go' and could run and jump and sleep and everything.

But, deep down inside in that place that some men will bury the things they don't want to admit to, I knew I had probably done a bit more than just bruise my hip - and my pride. That hip was always stiff and after long walks it ached. Occasionally it would get a bit stuck and took a moment to loosen up. At night it would throb a little.

I developed a keen interest in problems affecting the young adult hip and learned how to do keyhole surgery on the hip joint, which was a new technique considered too difficult to be very popular among most of my colleagues. I noticed that my patients would complain about very similar symptoms to those I was experiencing, and often they didn't appear to be in as much trouble as I was.

I did wonder if I should have an x-ray but I told myself that if I did, and it showed that I had in fact damaged my hip in 1996, and that it had now developed into osteoarthritis, it would probably just make it hurt more. It wasn't as if I needed an operation, no way was it bad enough for that. Was it?

Eventually, in early 2021, my good friend and colleague Richard Hargrove told me in no uncertain terms that I should bloody well have an x-ray and just admit I had a problem. He said that if I needed a hip replacement, he didn't want it to get so bad that he would have trouble giving me a decent result.

It turned out that my hip was rather worse than I had expected. I'd go as far to say that I would *never* have let a patient get that bad without strongly advising them to have a replacement.

Well, I had my new hip later that year, and it was only afterwards that I truly realised how much pain I had been in before it was done, such is the capacity for the musculo-skeletal system to adapt around a slowly deteriorating joint.

And the capacity for self-deception of some people who *should* know better.

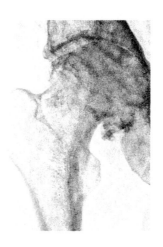

Maybe I shouldn't have waited *quite* so long?

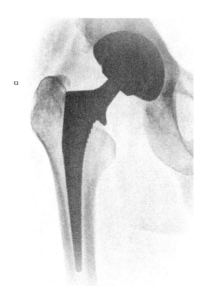

Nice result though!

Acknowledgements

I am indebted to Louise McOvens for her generous foreword and for showing us all how to survive despite everything.

To my many colleagues, friends and relatives who made suggestions and comments that have made this collection hopefully more readable, I am most grateful.

I could not have been the doctor I am in these stories without the love and support of my wife Lorraine. She has always had my back, helping me through the sad times as well as celebrating the wins.

Ultimately I must thank the patients, most of whom will never read these stories. It was my privilege to try and help you where I could.

Magic Daisy Publishing is an independent imprint which supports authors and illustrators who are interested in becoming published.

We'd love you to check out our website:

www.magicdaisypublishing.co.uk

If you have any feedback or would like to get in touch then you can email us:

magicdaisypublishing@outlook.com

You can also find us on Facebook where we have more information about our authors, illustrators and future competitions.

www.facebook.com/magicdaisypublishing

Thank you for your interest in Magic Daisy Publishing!

Magic
Daisy

Printed in Great Britain
by Amazon

39223559R00056